HOW TO BUID A WORKOUT ROUTINE

THE NEWBIES GUIDE

KATE .P

Contents

CHAPTER ONE

INTRODUCTION

Whether your objective is to increase overall health and endurance, shed pounds, or build muscle, developing a successful exercise regimen is crucial to reaching your fitness objectives. In addition to keeping you organized, a structured training program makes sure you're appropriately addressing various muscle groups and allowing for optimum recovery. Here's a basic overview of creating an exercise regimen:

Establish Specific Objectives: Decide what you hope to accomplish during your training. Your objectives will determine how your program is organized, whether they be to increase flexibility, lose weight, build strength, or improve cardiovascular health.

Evaluate Your Fitness Level: Creating a program that challenges you correctly without putting you at risk for injury requires that you have a clear understanding of your current fitness level. Evaluate your flexibility, strength, endurance, and any particular weak points.

Choose Your Exercises: Make sure the workouts you choose fit your goals and your interests. This could involve working on your flexibility, strength, or cardiovascular fitness, or a mix of these. Adding variety to your workouts keeps them engaging and helps you avoid monotony.

Make a schedule for yourself by deciding how many days a week and how long each workout will last. Take into account things like employment, family responsibilities, and other commitments when estimating how much time you can dedicate.

Maintain a Balance in Your Routine: Make sure your regimen consists of a variety of exercises that target different muscle groups and fitness levels. Aim for a balance between strength training, cardiovascular activity, and flexibility exercises.

Include a Warm-Up and Cool-Down: To get your body ready for exercise and lower your chance of injury, warm up properly before beginning any workout. In a similar vein, cool down at the end to gradually reduce heart rate and lengthen your muscles.

Progression and Variation: As your fitness level rises, progressively increase the volume, duration, or frequency of your workouts. Change up your workout from time to time to avoid plateaus and to continue pushing your body.

Listen to Your Body: Keep an eye on how exercise affects your physical composition. If you feel pain or discomfort, adjust your regimen or consult a fitness expert for guidance.

Remain Consistent: Observing results requires consistency. Make every effort to adhere to your exercise regimen, especially on the days when you lack motivation.

Rest and Recovery: To avoid overtraining and to encourage muscle growth and repair, give your body time to rest and recuperate in between sessions. Make leisure days a part of your schedule and give adequate rest and nourishment a high priority.

Creating an exercise program is a dynamic process that may need to be adjusted as your goals, preferences, and progress change. Try out various workouts and regimens to determine what suits you the best, and don't be afraid to ask fitness experts for advice if you need it. You may design an exercise regimen that will help you achieve your fitness goals if you are committed and persistent.

The value of a regimented exercise program

A well-planned exercise regimen is essential for a number of reasons, all of which help you achieve your fitness objectives and maximize the efficiency of your workouts:

Progression and Achieving Your Goals: With a regimented exercise program, you may gradually strain your cardiovascular system and muscles. Through incremental increases in workout intensity, length, or frequency, you may consistently push your body to reach new levels of fitness.

Efficiency: Making the most of your time in the gym or during your workouts is certain when you have a strategy. A set schedule helps you stay focused and effective rather than hopping around from workout to workout.

Balanced Development: All the main muscle groups and components of fitness strength, cardiovascular endurance, flexibility, and mobility are worked out in a well-planned program. This well-rounded strategy lowers the chance of overuse injuries and musculoskeletal imbalances while promoting general health.

Prevention of Plateaus: Including variation and growth in your routine can help you avoid hitting a wall when it comes to your fitness goals. When your body adjusts to your current exercise regimen, you hit a plateau and your development becomes stagnate. You can keep your body guessing and continue to make progress by switching up your workouts, rep ranges, and intensity levels on a regular basis.

Injury Prevention: Carefully designed programming takes into account variables such as recuperation, volume, intensity, and kind of exercise. You can lessen your chance of overuse injuries brought on by repetitive motions or high exercise volume by adhering to a regimen. Including mobility exercises, cool-downs, and warm-ups also helps your body get ready for exercise and reduces the chance of injury.

Accountability and Consistency: It's simpler to remain accountable for your exercise objectives when you have a set timetable and plan. Long-term improvement requires consistency in your workouts, which is more likely to occur when you know what's expected of you each day.

Personalization: An organized program can be made to meet your fitness level, interests, and desired outcomes. You can modify your workouts to suit your goals, whether they want to gain muscle mass, reduce body fat, increase overall health, or improve athletic performance.

Psychological Benefits: Sticking to a regimen gives you a sense of control and organization, which helps lessen the tension and worry that comes with working out. Furthermore, attaining objectives and observing improvement increases confidence and drive, which strengthens your will to stay fit.

All things considered, a planned exercise program acts as a road map for achievement, directing you toward your fitness objectives while lowering the possibility of obstacles or accidents. You may optimize your results and have a stronger, more resilient, and healthier physique by adhering to a carefully thought-out plan and maintaining consistency.

benefits of sticking to a regular exercise schedule

There are several advantages to sticking to a regular exercise schedule that improve mental and physical health:

Progress Towards Objectives: Whether your goal is to gain more muscle, lose weight, increase endurance, or improve your general health, consistency is essential to achieving your fitness objectives. Over time, consistent exercise improves cardiovascular health, increases metabolism, and promotes muscle growth.

Improved Strength and Endurance: Muscular strength and endurance increase with regular exercise. Resistance training is a great way to constantly challenge your muscles, which increases muscular growth and force production. Similar to this, cardiovascular exercises enhance lung and heart health, reducing fatigue during physical activity.

Weight management: By boosting metabolism and burning calories, regular exercise helps control body weight. Regular physical activity can help with weight loss or maintenance by generating a calorie deficit when paired with a balanced diet.

Enhanced Mental and Mood States: Physical activity triggers the release of endorphins, which are happy-making neurotransmitters. Regular exercise has been demonstrated to improve mental clarity and cognitive function while lowering stress, anxiety, and depressive symptom levels.

Enhanced Energy: Exercise on a regular basis enhances oxygen delivery to tissues and circulation, which raises energy levels and lessens weariness. Regular exercise can gradually increase your stamina and endurance, making it easier for you to carry out daily chores.

Increased Sleep Duration and Quality: Frequent exercise can extend and enhance sleep. Exercise facilitates relaxation and aids in the regulation of circadian rhythms, which makes it simpler to fall asleep and stay asleep through the night.

Lower Risk of Chronic Illness: Regular exercise has been linked to a lower risk of long-term illnesses like heart disease, type 2 diabetes, and several cancers. Frequent exercise strengthens the immune system, controls blood sugar, and enhances cardiovascular health—all of which help avoid disease.

Enhanced Self-Esteem and Confidence: Reaching fitness objectives and sticking to a regular exercise schedule can increase self-esteem and confidence.

CHAPTER TWO

Reaching goals like lifting bigger weights or finishing a difficult workout strengthens one's sense of accomplishment and value.

Social contact and Support: Regular attendance at fitness centers, group exercise sessions, or sporting events offers chances for social contact and support. Developing relationships with people who share your interests creates a sense of accountability and community, which helps you stay motivated and dedicated to your exercise regimen.

Long-Term Health and Longevity: Regular exercise is linked to a higher quality of life and longer longevity in older persons. Engaging in regular physical activity lowers the risk of falls, fractures, and age-related health problems by maintaining muscle mass, bone density, and mobility.

Maintaining a regular exercise schedule has many psychological, emotional, and physical advantages that enhance longevity and general well-being. One of the biggest things you can do to live a healthy, happy life is to incorporate exercise into your daily routine.

Evaluating Your Current Fitness Level and Your Fitness Goals

Identifying your fitness objectives and existing level of fitness is an essential first step in creating a successful training program. This is how you do it:

Establish Your Fitness Objectives: Give careful thought to the things you hope to accomplish with exercise. Your objectives can be to lose weight, grow muscle, increase flexibility, boost endurance, or focus on your general health and well-being. Ensure that your objectives are time-bound, meaningful, quantifiable, achievable, and specific (SMART).

Take Into Account Your Personal Preferences: Consider the kinds of activities you find enjoyable and are likely to engage in over time. Choosing fun activities for your exercise regimen enhances the likelihood that you will stay inspired and dedicated to it, whether it be jogging, weightlifting, swimming, yoga, or group fitness programs.

Determine Your Current Fitness Level: Consider your advantages, disadvantages, and starting point fitness level in a number of areas, such as:

Cardiovascular Endurance: The amount of time that you can engage in aerobic exercise, such as swimming, cycling, or running, without running out of breath?

Muscular Strength: What is your maximum weight capacity for different activities like bench presses, bicep curls, and squats?

Muscular Endurance: How many times can you complete a series of exercises without becoming fatigued?

Flexibility: How adaptable and supple are your joints and muscles? Can you properly do a deep squat or touch your toes?

Body Composition: What are your current measurements for muscle mass, body fat percentage, and weight? To determine your body composition, think about utilizing instruments like DEXA scans, body fat calipers, and body measurements.

Have Reasonable Expectations: Be truthful with yourself about your current situation and your realistic expectations for yourself. Unrealistic goals can cause dissatisfaction and fatigue.

Speak with Experts: If you're not sure how to evaluate your level of fitness or create realistic goals, think about getting advice from fitness specialists like registered dietitians, exercise physiologists, or personal trainers. They can offer professional guidance catered to your particular requirements and assist you in developing a customized strategy for success.

Track Your Progress: To keep yourself accountable and to keep an eye on your progress, keep a log of your workouts, measurements, and accomplishments throughout time. Maintaining a workout log, using fitness applications, or planning routine evaluations to gauge gains in strength, endurance, and other fitness metrics can all be easy ways to do this.

You can design an exercise regimen that is specific to your needs, tastes, and skills by carefully evaluating your fitness objectives and present level of fitness. It's important to keep in mind that maintaining your fitness level is a journey, so be patient and dedicated to your objectives.

Recognizing Various Exercise Types

Knowing the numerous exercise options accessible to you enables you to design a well-rounded fitness regimen that addresses multiple areas of fitness. The primary forms of exercise and its advantages are as follows:

Exercise for the Heart (Cardio):

Examples include jogging, riding, swimming, dancing, jumping rope, and fast walking.

Benefits include strengthening the heart and lungs to improve cardiovascular health, increasing stamina and endurance, burning calories to lose weight, lowering the risk of chronic diseases like diabetes and heart disease, elevating mood, and lowering stress.

Strengthening Exercise:

Examples include kettlebell workouts, resistance band exercises, bodyweight exercises including lunges, squats, and push-ups, and weightlifting.

Benefits include increased bone density, improved joint health and stability, improved muscular mass and strength, improved metabolism, assistance for weight management, improved sports performance, and decreased chance of injury.

Exercises for Flexibility and Mobility:

Examples include foam rolling, mobility drills, yoga, Pilates, and stretching.

Benefits include increased range of motion and flexibility, better posture and alignment of the body, lessened pain and tension in the muscles, improved athletic performance, less chance of injury, and encouragement of relaxation and stress alleviation.

Exercises for Stability and Balance:

Examples include balancing board exercises, stability ball exercises, Tai Chi, yoga, and single-leg workouts like single-leg squats.

Benefits include strengthening stabilizing muscles, increasing body awareness and proprioception, enhancing balance and coordination, lowering the risk of falls and accidents, and improving sports performance.

Practical Instruction:

Examples include kettlebell movements, TRX suspension training, and functional movement patterns like squats, lunges, pushing, and pulling.

Benefits include: improving total functional fitness and movement efficiency, improving sports performance, simulating real-life motions and activities, and lowering the chance of injury by strengthening muscles used in daily activities.

HIIT, or high-intensity interval training:

Exercises like Tabata, circuit training, interval jogging, and cycling sprints are some examples.

Benefits include: effective burning of fat and calories, enhancement of cardiovascular fitness, enhancement of metabolism for hours after exercise, preservation of muscle mass, enhancement of aerobic and anaerobic capacity, and time savings through shorter exercises.

Cross-Mission Training:

Examples: Including in your regimen a range of exercises from several modalities.

Benefits include preventing boredom and plateaus, lowering the chance of overuse injuries, increasing motivation and exercise adherence, and promoting general fitness and athleticism by testing various muscle groups and energy systems.

Including a mix of these workouts in your regimen guarantees overall fitness growth and lowers the chance of overuse issues. To maximize results and avoid burnout, customize your exercise regimen to meet your preferences, goals, and current level of fitness. Don't forget to incorporate enough time for rest and recovery as well.

Creating a Workout Program

Creating a training plan entails allocating scheduled, balanced time slots for your workouts each week. This is a step-by-step tutorial to assist you in making a productive exercise schedule:

Establish Realistic Goals: Identify your fitness objectives, including those pertaining to general health, muscular growth, weight loss, and endurance enhancement. The kind, frequency, and intensity of your planned workouts will depend on your goals.

Evaluate Your Availability: Take into account your weekly itinerary, taking into account your obligations to your family, job, and education.

Determine the days and times when you can consistently work out.

Select Your Workout Days: To ensure that you have enough time for rest and recuperation in between sessions, try to distribute your workouts evenly throughout the week. Most people find that, depending on their goals and availability, a routine consisting of three to five workout days per week works well.

Workout Duration: Choose the length of each workout based on your personal tastes, time limits, and fitness objectives. Depending on the sort and degree of exercise you plan to do, a workout might last anywhere from thirty minutes to an hour or more.

Choose Your Workout Modalities: Choose the workouts you'll perform in your regimen, such as cardio, strength, flexibility, or a mix of these. Make sure the activities on your schedule are well-balanced to target various muscle groups and fitness components.

Make Rest Days a Priority: To enable your body to heal and regenerate muscle tissue, plan at least one or two rest days every week. For the purpose of minimizing burnout and overtraining, rest days are equally as crucial as workout days.

Periodization is something to think about if you're on a regimented training program or have particular fitness objectives. Periodization can help you achieve both of these things. Periodization is breaking up your training into separate training phases, such as endurance, strength, or hypertrophy, each with a certain emphasis and degree of intensity.

Warm-up and Cool-down: Set aside time for warm-up exercises to get your body ready for exercise and lower your chance of injury before starting any workout. Likewise, incorporate a cool-down phase to gradually reduce heart rate and lengthen your muscles at the conclusion of your exercises.

While having a plan is important, it's also important to be adaptable and ready to change your schedule when necessary in response to things like exhaustion, soreness, or unforeseen circumstances. Additionally, pay attention to your body. Pay attention to your body and allow yourself to take breaks or adjust your exercise regimen as needed.

Track Your Progress: To keep track of your workouts, track your progress, and ensure that you are sticking to your program, keep a workout journal or use a fitness tracking app. In order to keep moving closer to your objectives, evaluate your performance on a regular basis and modify your routine or schedule as necessary.

Recall that the secret to achieving results is consistency, so make every effort to adhere to your exercise regimen. Creating a realistic, well-balanced fitness plan that fits your objectives and lifestyle can help you stay motivated, make progress, and get the rewards of consistent exercise.

A balanced fitness regimen should include a range of activities that focus on various muscle groups and fitness facets. Here's how to design a fitness program that is well-rounded:

Incorporate Strength Training: Include exercises that focus on important muscle groups, such as the arms, shoulders, back, legs, and chest. Aim for a well-rounded approach that incorporates pulling exercises (such as pull-ups and rows) and pushing exercises (such as shoulder presses and chest presses). Select challenging workouts that work multiple muscle groups at once, like lunges, deadlifts, and squats, in addition to isolation exercises that focus on particular muscle groups.

Include Cardiovascular Exercise: Incorporate heart-pumping, cardiovascular exercises to strengthen your heart. Exercises that are available include swimming, cycling, jogging, brisk walking, and aerobic dance classes. Every week, split up over several days, try to get in at least 150 minutes of moderate-intensity exercise or 75 minutes of vigorous-intensity cardio.

Make Flexibility and Mobility a Priority: Set aside time for mobility exercises and stretches to improve joint health, range of motion, and flexibility. Use static stretches to increase flexibility and reduce muscle tension after workouts and dynamic stretches to prime your muscles for movement. Think about doing Pilates, yoga, or foam rolling to increase range of motion and reduce the risk of injury.

Incorporate Core Work: To improve stability, posture, and overall functional strength, strengthen your core muscles, particularly the lower back, obliques, and abdominals. Incorporate core-attacking exercises from various perspectives, such as planks, Russian twists, bicycle crunches, and stability ball exercises.

Combine Balance and Stability Training: To enhance coordination and stability, include exercises that test your proprioception and balance. Exercises with a single leg, balance boards, stability balls, and functional motions that mimic everyday activities should all be included.

Change Up Your Routine: By making frequent adjustments to your routine, you can reduce plateaus and keep your workouts engaging. Every few weeks, switch up your exercises, sets, reps, and intensity levels to continuously challenge your body and prevent adaptation.

Progression: To maintain your progress, gradually increase the duration, intensity, or difficulty of your workouts over time. This could entail using heavier weights, stepping up the resistance, doing more sets or repetitions, or moving on to harder workouts.

Rest and Recovery: To avoid overtraining and promote muscle growth and repair, leave enough time between sessions for rest and recovery. Put rest days on your schedule and concentrate on getting enough rest, water, and food to aid in healing.

Listen to Your Body: Adjust your exercise routine based on how your body reacts to certain activities. Take a break or change your activities if you experience pain, tiredness, or extreme soreness to avoid further damage.

Seek Professional Advice: To create a training plan that is specifically tailored to your goals, fitness level, and any unique needs or limitations you may have, think about collaborating with a certified personal trainer or fitness coach.

You can create a well-rounded and effective training program that enhances general health, strength, endurance, flexibility, and functional fitness by incorporating these elements into your regimen. To keep moving closer to your fitness goals, never forget to be consistent, pay attention to your body, and make adjustments as necessary.

Selecting Workouts and Activities

The exercises and activities you select for your training program will depend on your current fitness level, preferences, and fitness goals. Here's how to locate exercises and pursuits that align with your goals:

Establish Your Objectives: Decide what you hope to accomplish with exercise. Your objectives will dictate the kinds of exercises you perform, whether they are to gain muscle, lose weight, enhance cardiovascular health, increase general fitness, or increase flexibility.

Think About Your Preferences: Choose workouts and pursuits that you find enjoyable and are likely to stick with over time. Selecting enjoyable activities for your fitness regimen, such as dancing, martial arts, weightlifting, swimming, yoga, jogging, or team sports, increases the likelihood that you will stick with it.

Evaluate Your Fitness Level: Consider your current level of fitness as well as any potential restrictions or limitations. Start with exercises that are suitable for your current level of strength, endurance, and flexibility if you're a beginner. Gradually advance to increasingly difficult maneuvers as you gain confidence and experience.

Select Functional Motions: To improve functional fitness and movement efficiency, include exercises that replicate motions and activities found in everyday life. Squats, lunges, deadlifts, push-ups, pull-ups, and overhead presses are a few examples. These compound movements improve overall athleticism and train a variety of muscle groups.

Include variety: To target different muscle groups and aspects of fitness, incorporate a variety of exercises and activities into your regimen. Build a well-rounded program that supports general health and fitness by incorporating functional movements, strength training, cardiovascular activity, and flexibility exercises.

Customize to Your Objectives: Choose workouts and pursuits that align with your own objectives. Prioritize compound exercises like squats, deadlifts, bench presses, and rows if your goal is to gain muscle. Combine calorie-burning activities such as cycling, jogging, or high-intensity interval training (HIIT) to lose weight. If you value flexibility, consider incorporating Pilates or yoga into your curriculum.

Think About Time and Equipment: Select workouts and pursuits based on your availability and schedule. Bodyweight exercises, resistance bands, and basic cardio routines like running or jumping rope can be great options if you're short on time or don't have access to equipment. On the other hand, you can diversify your regimen more if you have access to a gym or specialized equipment.

Listen to Your Body: Observe how various exercises and activities make you feel in your body. To avoid injury and overtraining, modify your routine if you experience pain, discomfort, or exhaustion. Pay close attention to your form and technique to ensure a safe and effective training experience.

Seek Advice from Experts: If you're not sure which workouts are best for your objectives or if you have particular health concerns, you should think about seeking advice from certified fitness instructors, personal trainers, or medical professionals. They can offer professional advice and create a personalized exercise plan based on your particular needs.

You can create an enjoyable, effective, and long-lasting fitness program by selecting exercises and activities that align with your goals, interests, and current level of fitness. Try out a variety of workouts and activities to see what suits you the best. Don't be afraid to make changes as necessary to keep your workouts interesting and demanding.

Organizing Exercises for Warm-Up and Cool-Down

It's essential to plan your warm-up and cool-down periods to get your body ready for exercise and help with recovery afterward. Here's how to efficiently organize both sessions:

Warm-Up Time:

Start with General Movements: To increase blood flow and raise your heart rate, start your warm-up with mild cardiovascular exercises. Running, brisk walking, cycling, and jumping jacks are a few examples. To gradually raise your body temperature, try low-intensity movement for five to ten minutes.

Dynamic Stretching: To improve range of motion and flexibility, incorporate dynamic stretches that focus on your main muscles and joints. Execute motions like hip circles, torso twists, leg swings, and arm circles. Stretching with movement helps activate muscles and gets them ready for harder training.

Workouts that target specific muscles or muscle groups that you'll use are a good way to activate your muscles. Bodyweight exercises like squats, lunges, push-ups, and band exercises may be a part of this. To encourage proper form and movement patterns, concentrate on using your core and stabilizing muscles.

Sport-specific Drills (Optional): Include drills or exercises that replicate the skills or motions required for the sport or activity you participate in. For instance, incorporate dynamic drills like leg swings, high knees, and butt kicks if you're getting ready for a run.

Increase Intensity Gradually: Raise the intensity of your warm-up gradually to correspond with the demands of your exercise. When your major workout approaches, gradually increase the intensity of the movements you're doing from a gentle start. Increased heart rate, improved blood flow to the muscles, and mental readiness for the exercise ahead are the goals.

Cool-down Period:

reduce Intensity: To help your heart rate return to baseline following your primary workout, progressively reduce the intensity of your activity. Change your workout from high-intensity to low-intensity exercises or static stretches.

Static Stretching: To target major muscle groups and improve flexibility, perform static stretches. Hold each stretch for 15–30 seconds, paying particular attention to tense or constricted areas. Particularly focus on the muscles in your quadriceps, hamstrings, calves, chest, back, and shoulders that were heavily worked during your workout.

Foam Rolling or Self-Myofascial Release: To release tension from muscles and fascia, use a foam roller or other massage instrument. Roll over tense or uncomfortable areas, applying light pressure to ease soreness in the muscles and improve tissue elasticity.

Deep Breathing and Relaxation: To help lower stress and speed up recovery, spend a few minutes concentrating on deep breathing and relaxation techniques. To calm the nerves and promote muscle relaxation, try diaphragmatic breathing or guided meditation.

Hydration and Nutrition: Consume a balanced post-workout meal or snack to replenish lost fluids and nutrients following physical activity. Try to consume a mix of protein and carbs to aid in muscle repair and replenish glycogen stores.

Think and Make Plans: Give your workout and your feelings during it some thought. Make a note of any areas that need work or adjustments you might need to make for next exercises. Make use of this time to set goals for your upcoming training sessions and schedule them appropriately.

CHAPTER THREE

Planned warm-up and cool-down sessions can improve performance, lower the risk of injury, and promote overall health and recovery when incorporated into your training program. Based on your individual fitness level and demands, as well as the length and intensity of your workouts, modify the length and intensity of your warm-up and cool-down.

A key component of fitness training is progression and adaptation, which entails gradually escalating the volume, intensity, or complexity of your workouts in order to promote ongoing gains in general fitness, strength, and endurance. Here's how to effectively incorporate progression and adaptability into your training regimen:

Gradual Progression: To help your body adjust and avoid damage, progression should be made gradually. Gradually and gradually increase the duration, intensity, or complexity of your workouts. Instead of making abrupt changes in intensity, strive for gradual, sustainable improvements over time.

Progressive Overload: Put this theory into practice by consistently pushing your cardiovascular system and muscles beyond their current comfort zones. This can be accomplished by increasing the resistance (lifting bigger weights, for example), the number of repetitions or sets, or the intensity of the cardiovascular exercise (running longer or faster, for example).

Variation: To avoid plateaus and promote ongoing progress, mix things up in your workouts. To keep your body challenged and prevent adaptation, switch up the exercises in your routine, try different training modalities (HIIT, circuit training, strength training, flexibility training, etc.), or rotate your workouts.

Periodization: Make deliberate adjustments to the volume and intensity of your training during specific intervals or cycles by using periodization. This may entail dividing your training program into distinct phases, each with a distinct emphasis and degree of intensity, such as hypertrophy, strength, power, or endurance. Periodization maximizes performance gains, encourages recovery, and reduces overtraining.

Rest and Recovery: Give adequate time to rest and recuperate so that your body can properly adjust to the stress of exercise. Incorporate days of rest into your routine, change up the volume and intensity of your workouts, and make sure you're getting enough rest, water, and food to help your body heal and adapt.

Listen to Your Body: Adjust your workout routines based on how your body reacts to training. In order to allow for the best possible recovery, you may need to reduce the volume or intensity of your workouts if you experience persistent fatigue, soreness, or decreased performance.

Establish Realistic Goals: To help you progress and stay motivated, set SMART (specific, measurable, achievable, relevant, and time-bound) goals. To maintain momentum and focus, break down larger goals into smaller benchmarks and recognize and celebrate your progress along the way.

Periodic Assessments: Evaluate your performance and progress on a regular basis to identify areas for improvement and track your progress. This could entail keeping track of body measurements, tracking the amount of weight lifted, measuring workout length or distance, or evaluating fitness benchmarks (e.g., one-rep max, mile time). Make use of these evaluations to inform your training decisions and adjust your workout regimen as necessary.

Maintaining consistency is essential for long-term success and adaptation. Maintain your training schedule, especially on days when you're not feeling very motivated. Consistency is more important than perfection. Recall that progress takes time, and maintaining your commitment to your fitness objectives will pay off in the long run.

You can effectively promote adaptation and continuous development in your fitness journey by incorporating progressive overload, variation, periodization, and recovery tactics into your training regimen. As you work toward your objectives, exercise patience, maintain focus, and have faith in the process.

Including Rest and Recuperation

It is essential to include rest and recovery into your exercise routine in order to maximize results, minimize overtraining, and preserve long-term health and fitness. Here's how to effectively fit rest and recuperation into your schedule:

regular Rest Days: Schedule specific rest days into your weekly training regimen to give your body the time it needs to recover and mend. Aim for one or two rest days per week, based on your level of fitness, training volume, and specific needs for recovery.

Listen to Your Body: Be aware of any cues your body is giving you, such as fatigue, pain, decreased function, or recurrent injuries. To allow for the best possible recovery, if you're feeling too exhausted or worn out, think about taking an extra day off or reducing the frequency and intensity of your workouts.

Active Recovery: To improve blood flow, reduce muscle stiffness, and speed up recovery, include light or low-intensity exercise on rest days.

Walking, gentle yoga, swimming, cycling, and other activities can help reduce stiffness and soreness without putting undue strain on your joints and muscles.

Make sleep a priority because it's an essential part of rehabilitation. Try to get 7–9 hours of uninterrupted sleep every night to help with hormone regulation, muscle repair, and general physical and mental health. Make changes to your sleeping environment, establish a nightly routine, and limit your exposure to electronics and stimulating activities right before bed.

Nutrition and Hydration: To aid in healing and restock energy storage, fuel your body with healthful foods and the right amount of water. Eat a well-balanced diet high in healthy fats, carbohydrates, protein, and vitamins and minerals to support muscle repair and glycogen resupply. Drink water to stay hydrated throughout the day, particularly before, during, and after physical activity.

Foam Rolling and Mobility Work: To ease tense muscles, increase range of motion, and accelerate healing, include foam rolling, self-myofascial release, and mobility exercises in your routine. To improve tissue quality and release knots and adhesions, spend some time using a foam roller, massage ball, or mobility tools to target tight or uncomfortable areas.

Stretching and Flexibility Training: To improve range of motion, lessen muscle stiffness, and avoid injury, incorporate static stretching and flexibility exercises. To promote relaxation and speed up recovery, stretch your major muscle groups after working out or as part of your cool-down routine.

Massage & Bodywork: To address musculoskeletal imbalances, relieve tension, and promote relaxation, think about incorporating bodywork techniques like chiropractic therapy, professional massage, or other bodywork methods into your recovery program. Frequent massages can enhance general wellbeing, hasten healing, and improve circulation.

Mental and Emotional Recovery: To lower stress hormones and improve mental and emotional recovery, practice stress-reduction techniques like deep breathing, mindfulness, and meditation.

Aside from exercising, make time for relaxation, rest, and enjoyment of your favorite hobbies.

Periodic Deloads: To reduce overtraining and allow for supercompensation, schedule deload weeks or periods of lowered training volume and intensity every 4-6 weeks. Reduce the frequency, length, or intensity of your workouts during deloads to give your body a rest while keeping your activity levels the same.

Including strategies for rest and recovery into your training regimen can help you reach your fitness objectives over the long term, perform better, and experience less burnout. To promote general health and well-being, make self-care a priority, pay attention to your body's needs, and find a balance between exercise and relaxation.

Maintaining Consistency and Motivation

Achieving your fitness objectives and sustaining long-term success in your training program depend heavily on your motivation and persistence. The following techniques will support you in maintaining your commitment to your fitness journey:

Establish Specific and Attainable Objectives: Identify exciting and motivating goals that are specific, quantifiable, and achievable. Having specific goals gives your training focus and direction, whether it's losing weight, finishing a 5k, or increasing strength in particular lifts.

Break Big Goals Down into More Manageable Milestones: To monitor your progress and recognize accomplishments along the way, break big goals down into more manageable milestones. Establishing reasonable benchmarks promotes motivation and a feeling of accomplishment as you advance toward your ultimate goal.

Discover Your Why: Determine the reasons behind your desire to maintain your health and fitness. Understanding your underlying motivations can help you stay focused and committed when faced with challenges, whether they are related to enhancing your physical health, lowering stress, increasing confidence, or setting a positive example for others.

Establish a Consistent Routine: Make an effort to maintain your regular exercise schedule. To create habits and incorporate exercise into your daily routine, you must be consistent. Make time for exercise a priority and regard it as an appointment that you cannot miss.

Mix Up Your Workouts: Add variation to your routine to make your workouts engaging and fascinating. To keep yourself motivated and avoid boredom, experiment with different workouts, check out new clubs or activities, and switch up your schedule frequently.

Choose Exercises and Activities You Enjoy: Make a list of the things you genuinely enjoy and look forward to doing each day. Finding activities that you enjoy doing, whether it's dancing, hiking, sports, or weightlifting, will help you stay motivated and dedicated over time.

Workout with a Friend or Partner: To increase social support and accountability for your routine, work out with a workout partner or enroll in group fitness classes. Exercise can be more fun when done with a friend or partner, and it can also motivate you to show up and give it your all.

Track Your Progress: To stay motivated and see your progress, keep a record of your workouts, accomplishments, and progress. Track your progress, celebrate your victories, and keep track of your workouts with a fitness journal, app, or wearable fitness tracker.

Reward Yourself: Create a system of rewards to encourage regularity and devotion to your exercise regimen. When you accomplish a goal or reach a milestone, treat yourself to something enjoyable or meaningful, like a day off, a massage, or a new workout attire.

Remain Upbeat and Adaptable: Adopt a growth mindset and concentrate on the advantages of physical activity. Acknowledge that obstacles and disappointments are a normal part of the journey and be willing to change course when necessary. Continue to be positive, take lessons from failures, and advance with tenacity and fortitude.

You can overcome challenges, keep your motivation high, and reap the long-term rewards of an active, healthy lifestyle by putting these strategies into practice and remaining dedicated to your fitness objectives.

Any fitness journey will inevitably involve challenges. However, by learning how to troubleshoot and overcome common obstacles, you can stay on track and accomplish your goals. The following are some methods for resolving typical issues with your exercise regimen:

Lack of motivation:

Remind yourself of your objectives and motivations for working out.

Divide your objectives into more manageable, smaller milestones.

Look for things to do that you truly look forward to and enjoy.

To keep yourself accountable, ask friends, family, or a workout partner for support.

Try out different exercises, programs, or regimens to keep things interesting and novel.

Time Limitations:

Make fitness a priority by incorporating workouts into your weekly or daily schedule.

When you are short on time, choose high-intensity, shorter workouts.

If needed, divide up your workouts into shorter bursts throughout the day.

To cut down on travel time, opt for activities that can be completed at home or with little equipment.

Standstill:

Adapt your training modalities, intensity levels, and exercises to make your workouts more interesting.

To push your body further, try increasing the duration or intensity of your workouts.

Make periodization a part of your regimen by alternating between training phases.

To increase productivity and outcomes, concentrate on honing form and technique.

Seek advice from a fitness specialist for individualized direction and planning.

Pain or Injury:

Pay attention to your body's needs and refrain from ignoring pain or discomfort.

Exercise modifications or low-impact substitutions can help prevent injuries from getting worse.

To avoid injuries, include active recovery days, rest days, and appropriate warm-up and cool-down routines in your exercise regimen.

If you have ongoing pain or discomfort, see a healthcare provider for a diagnosis, treatment, and rehabilitation.

Absence of Advancement

To make sure your goals are reasonable and attainable, reevaluate them and make any necessary adjustments.

Analyze your sleeping, eating, drinking, and stress-reduction practices to find possible areas for improvement.

Keep track of your exercises, development, and performance to spot trends and areas in which you can improve.

Get input from a trainer, coach, or other qualified fitness specialist to pinpoint problem areas and hone your strategy.

Lack of Interest or Variety:

To keep things fresh, try out new sports, courses, or training regimens.

Establish short-term objectives or challenges to give yourself excitement and a sense of purpose.

Experiment with different training modalities, equipment, and exercises to add variety to your workouts.

Include sports, leisure activities, or outdoor pursuits in your routine to make it more enjoyable and varied.

Stress or Problems with Mental Health:

Make self-care and stress-reduction methods like mindfulness exercises, deep breathing, and meditation a priority.

Exercise can be used as an emotional release and stress reliever.

If you find yourself having trouble managing stress, anxiety, or depression, get help from friends, family, or mental health professionals.

Depending on your energy and emotional state, modify the intensity or focus of your workout, and remember to treat yourself with kindness when things get tough.

You can overcome obstacles, maintain motivation, and keep moving closer to your fitness goals by putting these strategies into practice and taking proactive measures to address common challenges. To succeed over the long term in your fitness journey, keep in mind that consistency, patience, and resilience are essential.

Starting a fitness journey has many positive effects on the body, mind, and soul. It is a life-changing experience. We've covered a lot of ground in this guide when it comes to creating an effective workout regimen, such as the value of structure, determining fitness objectives and levels, choosing suitable workouts, factoring in rest and recovery, and resolving typical problems. You may design a sustainable, well-balanced fitness program that meets your personal goals by putting these ideas and tactics to use.

It's critical to keep in mind that improving your fitness is a journey rather than a destination, and that success frequently happens in tiny, gradual steps. The most important qualities to develop along the road are perseverance, patience, and consistency. Accept the journey, acknowledge your accomplishments, and draw lessons from failures. Remain flexible, pay attention to your health, and keep an open mind to fresh chances for development.

Any fitness endeavor's ultimate goal is to improve general health, vitality, and well-being so that you can live a more active and satisfying life. The first step towards improved health can be taking up strength training, endurance training, weight loss, or just making self-care a priority. Now is the time to take action and let your dedication to fitness lead the way to a better, healthier future.

May the pursuit of excellence bring you joy, may your challenges give you strength, and may your daily progress bring you fulfillment as you continue on your fitness journey. Never forget that you have the ability to control your destiny and build the life you want. Cheers to your well-being, joy, and accomplishments in all your fitness pursuits. Continue onward, and may your path be paved with courage, resiliency, and endless opportunities.

THE END